BEAT COLORECTAL CANCER

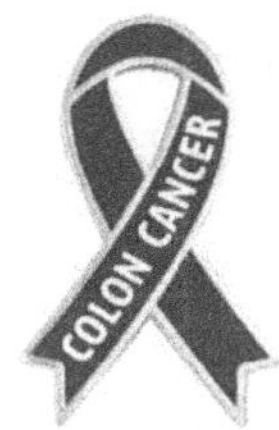

The Ultimate Guide On How To Fight Colorectal Cancer Using The Best Of Natural Remedies And Modern Medicines

SHARON AMY

Table of contents

Introduction 4

Overview of colorectal cancer 5

Chapter 1: Understanding Colorectal Cancer 7

What is Colorectal Cancer? 7

Causes and Risk Factors 8

Symptoms and Warning Signs 11

Diagnosis and Staging 13

Types of Colorectal Cancer 15

Genetic and Familial Factors 18

Chapter 2: Prevention and Screening 23

Importance of Screening 23

Screening Tests 25

Screening Guidelines and Recommendations 27

Lifestyle Modifications for   Prevention 30

Hereditary Syndromes and Screening
Recommendations 32

Chapter 3: Treatment Options 35

Treatment Overview: Surgery, Chemotherapy,
Radiation Therapy 35

Surgical Approaches: Colectomy, Laparoscopic
Surgery, Robotic Surgery 38

Chemotherapy: Drugs, Side Effects, and
Management 42

Radiation Therapy: Techniques and Side
Effects 46

Targeted Therapy and   Immunotherapy 49

Clinical Trials and Experimental Treatments 53

Chapter 4: Living with Colorectal Cancer 59

Coping with Diagnosis and Treatment 59

Nutritional Guidance During Treatment 62

Managing Side Effects: Fatigue, Nausea, Diarrhea, Neuropathy 68

Emotional and Psychological Support 71

Integrative Therapies: Acupuncture, Massage, Yoga 75

Sexual Health and Fertility Concerns 78

Support for Caregivers and Loved Ones 82

Chapter 5: Survivorship and Beyond 86

Life After Treatment: Follow-Up Care and Surveillance 87

Late and Long-Term Effects of Treatment 94

Recurrence: Signs, Symptoms, and Management 98

Advocacy and Resources for Patients and Survivors 102

Inspiring Stories of Survival 106

Conclusion 110

Hope and Future Directions in Colorectal Cancer Research 111

Introduction

Overview of colorectal cancer

Colorectal cancer is a type of cancer that affects the colon or rectum. Early cases can begin as non-cancerous polyps, which can turn into cancer over time. Once colon cancer has developed, it may still be years before it is detected. This process may occur over many years without producing any symptoms, but can be detected by screening. For this reason, doctors recommend screenings for those at high risk or over the age of 50. Colorectal cancer is the third most common cancer diagnosed in both men and women in the U.S, excluding skin cancers. While overall rates of people being diagnosed with colorectal cancer have decreased each year, young people are developing colorectal cancer at higher rates than ever before.

Because of this, the American Cancer Society lowered the recommended screening age in 2021 from 50 to 45 years old. Early detection through screenings like colonoscopies is key for successful treatment. Nutrition also plays a critical role in prevention and treatment. The foods you consume and the lifestyle you lead impact your cancer risk levels and your body's ability to prevent cancer. Some cancer research studies have found that people who eat right, get regular physical activity, maintain a healthy weight and limit alcohol consumption can cut their odds of colorectal disease by more than a third.

Remember, it's always best to consult with a healthcare professional for personalized advice and guidance, and also learn what foods to choose or lose to achieve a balanced diet for colorectal cancer prevention, plus dietary guidelines to follow during treatment.

This book is a source of inspiration to many on their path to healing, with this book you get a newfound appreciation for life and a desire to help others facing similar challenges.

Chapter 1: Understanding Colorectal Cancer

What is Colorectal Cancer?

Colorectal cancer, also known as colon cancer or rectal cancer, is a type of cancer that starts in the colon or rectum, which are parts of the large intestine. It typically develops from abnormal growths called polyps that form on the inner lining of the colon or rectum. Over time, some polyps may become cancerous.

Colorectal cancer is one of the most common types of cancer worldwide, with risk factors including age, family history, genetics, lifestyle factors such as diet and physical activity, and certain medical conditions like inflammatory bowel disease. Symptoms of colorectal cancer may include changes in bowel habits, blood in the stool, abdominal discomfort or pain, unexplained weight loss, and fatigue.

Early detection through screening tests such as colonoscopy, fecal occult blood test (FOBT), or flexible sigmoidoscopy can help detect colorectal cancer in its early stages when treatment is most effective. Treatment options for colorectal cancer may include surgery, chemotherapy, radiation therapy, targeted therapy, and immunotherapy, depending on the stage and characteristics of the cancer.

Overall, colorectal cancer is a serious but often treatable condition, especially when detected early. It's essential for individuals to be aware of risk factors, undergo recommended screenings, and seek medical attention if they experience any symptoms suggestive of colorectal cancer.

Causes and Risk Factors

The causes of colon cancer are multifactorial, involving a combination of genetic, environmental, and lifestyle factors. Here's a breakdown of the primary causes:

Genetic Factors: Certain genetic mutations can predispose individuals to colon cancer. Inherited conditions such as familial adenomatous polyposis (FAP) and hereditary nonpolyposis colorectal cancer (HNPCC), also known as Lynch syndrome, significantly increase the risk of developing colon cancer.

Family History: Having a close relative, such as a parent, sibling, or child, who has had colon cancer increases an individual's risk of developing the disease. The risk is higher if multiple family members are affected or if the relative was diagnosed at a young age.

Age: The risk of colon cancer increases with age, with the majority of cases diagnosed in individuals over the age of 50. However, colon cancer can occur at any age.

Polyps: Colorectal polyps are abnormal growths that can develop in the lining of the colon or rectum. While most polyps are benign, some may progress to cancer over time. Adenomatous polyps (adenomas) are the most common type of polyps that can develop into colon cancer.

Inflammatory Bowel Diseases (IBD): Chronic inflammation of the colon, as seen in conditions such as ulcerative colitis and Crohn's disease, increases the risk of developing colon cancer over time.

Dietary Factors: Diets high in red and processed meats, low in fiber, fruits, and vegetables, and high in saturated fats have been linked to an increased risk of colon cancer. Consumption of alcohol and sugary beverages may also contribute to the development of the disease.

Lifestyle Choices: Lack of physical activity, obesity, smoking, and excessive alcohol consumption have been identified as risk factors for colon cancer. These lifestyle choices can promote inflammation and other processes that contribute to cancer development.

Diabetes: Individuals with type 2 diabetes have an increased risk of developing colon cancer, although the exact mechanisms underlying this association are not fully understood.

Radiation Therapy: Previous exposure to radiation therapy for other cancers, particularly in the abdominal or pelvic area, can increase the risk of developing colon cancer later in life.

Environmental Factors: Exposure to certain environmental toxins, pollutants, and industrial chemicals may also contribute to the development of colon cancer, although the evidence is less well-established compared to other risk factors.

RISK FACTORS

Overall, the lifetime risk of developing colorectal cancer is about one in 23 for men and one in 26 for women. However, each person's risk might be higher or lower depending on their risk factors.

These may include:

• Being overweight or obese

• Low physical activity

• Diet

• Smoking

• Alcohol use

• Age

• Personal or family history of colorectal polyps or colorectal cancer

• Pre-existing conditions

• Racial or ethnic background

The American Cancer Society recommends that individuals at average risk begin regular screening at 45 years old.

Symptoms and Warning Signs

The symptoms of colon cancer can vary depending on the location of the tumor, its size, and how far it has spread. Some common symptoms and warning signs of colon cancer include:

Changes in Bowel Habits: Persistent changes in bowel habits, such as diarrhea, constipation, or changes in stool consistency, may indicate colon cancer.

Blood in the Stool: Blood in the stool can be bright red or dark and tarry, and it may be visible in the stool or on toilet paper. While not always a sign of colon cancer, it should be evaluated by a healthcare professional.

Abdominal Discomfort or Pain: Persistent abdominal pain, cramping, or discomfort, especially if it's accompanied by bloating or gas, may be a symptom of colon cancer.

Unexplained Weight Loss: Significant and unexplained weight loss, especially if it occurs rapidly without changes in diet or exercise, can be a warning sign of colon cancer.

Fatigue: Persistent fatigue or weakness that doesn't improve with rest may be a symptom of colon cancer, especially if it's accompanied by other symptoms.

Incomplete Emptying of Bowel: Feeling that your bowel doesn't completely empty after a bowel movement, or a feeling of fullness or blockage in the rectum, may indicate a tumor blocking the colon.

Iron Deficiency Anemia: Low levels of red blood cells (anemia) due to chronic blood loss from the colon can lead to symptoms such as fatigue, weakness, and pale skin.

Nausea or Vomiting: Persistent nausea or vomiting, especially if it's accompanied by other symptoms, may indicate a blockage in the colon caused by a tumor.

Changes in Appetite: Loss of appetite or feeling full quickly, even after eating small amounts of food, may be a symptom of colon cancer.

It's important to note that these symptoms can also be caused by other, less serious conditions such as hemorrhoids, irritable bowel syndrome (IBS), or inflammatory bowel disease (IBD). However, if you experience any persistent or concerning symptoms, especially if they persist for more than a few weeks, it's essential to see a healthcare professional for evaluation.

Diagnosis and Staging

The diagnosis and staging of colon cancer involve several steps to determine the extent of the disease and guide treatment decisions. Here's an overview of the process:

Diagnosis:

Medical History and Physical Examination: The healthcare provider will take a detailed medical history and perform a physical examination to assess symptoms and risk factors for colon cancer.
Diagnostic Tests:
•**Colonoscopy:** A colonoscopy is the gold standard for diagnosing colon cancer. During this procedure, a flexible tube with a camera is inserted into the

colon to visualize the lining and detect any abnormalities, such as polyps or tumors. Biopsies may be taken during the procedure for further evaluation.

•**Flexible Sigmoidoscopy:** Similar to a colonoscopy, but it only examines the lower part of the colon (sigmoid colon) and rectum.

•**Imaging Studies:** Imaging tests such as CT scans, MRI scans, or PET scans may be performed to evaluate the extent of the cancer and determine if it has spread to other parts of the body.

Laboratory Tests: Blood tests may be conducted to assess levels of certain markers, such as carcinoembryonic antigen (CEA), which may be elevated in individuals with colon cancer.

Staging:

Once a diagnosis of colon cancer is confirmed, staging is performed to determine the extent of the disease. The most commonly used staging system for colon cancer is the TNM staging system, which evaluates:

Tumor (T): The size and extent of the primary tumor.

Lymph Nodes (N): Whether the cancer has spread to nearby lymph nodes.

Metastasis (M): Whether the cancer has spread to distant organs or tissues.

Based on these factors, colon cancer is typically staged from 0 to IV:

•**Stage 0:** Also known as carcinoma in situ, the cancer is confined to the inner lining of the colon or rectum.
•**Stage I:** The cancer has grown into the deeper layers of the colon or rectum but has not spread beyond the wall of the organ.
•**Stage II:** The cancer has spread beyond the wall of the colon or rectum but has not yet reached nearby lymph nodes.
•**Stage III:** The cancer has spread to nearby lymph nodes but has not spread to distant organs.
•**Stage IV:** The cancer has spread to distant organs or tissues, such as the liver, lungs, or peritoneum.

Treatment Planning:

Once the stage of the colon cancer is determined, healthcare providers can develop a treatment plan tailored to the individual's specific needs. Treatment options may include surgery, chemotherapy, radiation therapy, targeted therapy, immunotherapy, or a combination of these approaches. The goal of treatment is to remove the cancer, prevent its recurrence, and improve overall survival and quality of life.

Types of Colorectal Cancer

Colorectal cancer can be categorized into different types based on various factors such as the location of the cancer within the colon or rectum, the histological characteristics of the tumor cells, and genetic mutations. These are some common types of colorectal cancer:

Adenocarcinoma: This is the most common type of colorectal cancer, accounting for over 95% of cases. Adenocarcinomas develop from the cells that line the inner surface of the colon and rectum. They typically start as benign growths called adenomatous polyps, which can eventually become cancerous.

Mucinous Adenocarcinoma: This subtype of adenocarcinoma is characterized by the presence of mucin, a gel-like substance, within the tumor cells. Mucinous adenocarcinomas may have a different appearance under the microscope and may behave differently than typical adenocarcinomas.

Signet Ring Cell Carcinoma: Signet ring cell carcinoma is a rare and aggressive type of colorectal cancer characterized by tumor cells with a distinctive signet ring appearance when viewed under a microscope. These cells contain abundant mucin, and the tumors tend to be more aggressive and have a poorer prognosis compared to other types of colorectal cancer.

Serrated Adenocarcinoma: Serrated adenocarcinomas arise from serrated polyps, which have a distinct appearance under the microscope. These tumors are associated with certain genetic mutations and may have different clinical and pathological characteristics compared to traditional adenocarcinomas.

Lymphoma: Lymphoma is a type of cancer that originates in the lymphatic system, but it can occasionally involve the colon or rectum. Colorectal lymphomas are rare and may present with symptoms similar to other types of colorectal cancer.

Neuroendocrine Tumors: Neuroendocrine tumors, also known as carcinoid tumors, can develop in the colon or rectum. These tumors arise from neuroendocrine cells and can be classified as well-differentiated or poorly differentiated based on their appearance and behavior.

Gastrointestinal Stromal Tumors (GISTs): GISTs are rare tumors that can develop in the gastrointestinal tract, including the colon and rectum. These tumors arise from specialized cells called interstitial cells of Cajal and may have different treatment approaches compared to other types of colorectal cancer.

These are the primary types of colorectal cancer, but there may be additional subtypes or variations based on specific molecular or genetic characteristics. Treatment decisions are often based on the type, stage, and other individual factors of the cancer.

Genetic and Familial Factors

Genetic and familial factors play a significant role in the development of colon cancer. Here's an overview of some of the key genetic and familial factors associated with colon cancer:

Hereditary Syndromes:

•**Familial Adenomatous Polyposis (FAP):** FAP is an inherited condition characterized by the development of hundreds to thousands of colorectal polyps in the colon and rectum, usually starting in the teenage years. Individuals with FAP have a nearly 100% risk of developing colorectal cancer if untreated.

•Hereditary Nonpolyposis Colorectal Cancer (HNPCC), also known as Lynch Syndrome: Lynch syndrome is caused by inherited mutations in genes responsible for DNA repair, such as MLH1, MSH2, MSH6, PMS2, and EPCAM. Individuals with Lynch syndrome have an increased risk of developing colorectal cancer, as well as other cancers including endometrial, ovarian, stomach, small intestine, pancreatic, and urinary tract cancers.

Family History:

•Having a first-degree relative (parent, sibling, or child) who has had colorectal cancer increases an individual's risk of developing the disease. The risk is higher if multiple family members are affected or if the relative was diagnosed at a young age.

•Individuals with a family history of adenomatous polyps or other colorectal conditions may also have an increased risk of developing colon cancer.

Genetic Mutations:

While hereditary syndromes like FAP and Lynch syndrome are caused by specific gene mutations, other genetic mutations can also contribute to the development of colon cancer. For example, mutations in genes such as APC, KRAS, BRAF, TP53, and SMAD4 have been associated with the development and progression of colorectal cancer.

Age: While not strictly genetic, age is a significant risk factor for colon cancer, and genetic factors may influence the risk of developing the disease as individuals age.

Environmental and Lifestyle Factors: While not directly inherited, certain environmental and lifestyle factors can interact with genetic predispositions to increase the risk of colon cancer. These factors include diet, physical activity, smoking, and alcohol consumption.

It's important to note that while genetic and familial factors can increase the risk of colon cancer, not everyone with these risk factors will develop the disease. Additionally, individuals without a family history of colon cancer can still develop the disease, and some cases of colon cancer occur without any known genetic predisposition. If you have concerns about your genetic or familial risk of colon cancer, it's best to discuss them with a healthcare provider or genetic counselor who can provide personalized risk assessment and recommendations for screening and prevention.

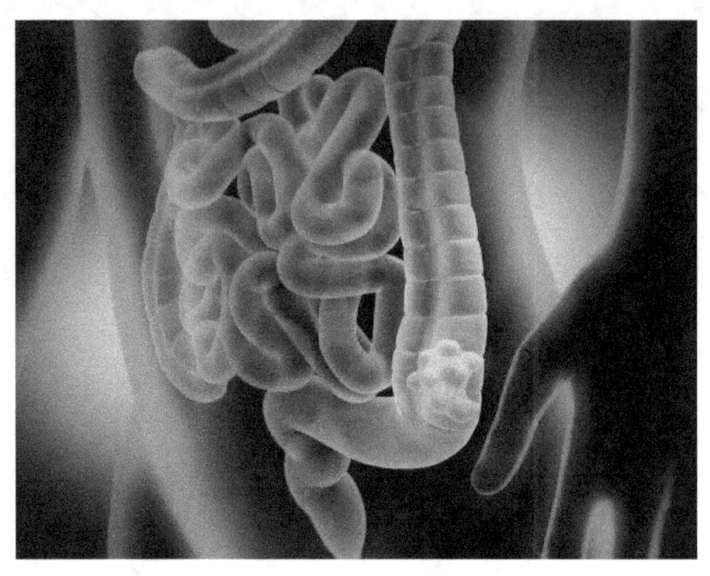

Chapter 2: Prevention and Screening

Importance of Screening

Screening for colon cancer is crucial for both individual health and public health. It's recommended that individuals discuss screening options with their healthcare provider, starting at age 50 for average-risk individuals, or earlier for those with certain risk factors or a family history of colon cancer. Early detection through screening can save lives and improve outcomes for individuals at risk of colon cancer. Here are some of the importance of screening;

Early Detection: Screening tests can detect colon cancer in its early stages, often before symptoms develop. When colon cancer is detected early, it's highly treatable, with better outcomes and a higher chance of cure.

Prevention: Certain screening tests, such as colonoscopy, can also help prevent colon cancer by identifying and removing precancerous growths called polyps before they have the chance to develop into cancer. This can significantly reduce the risk of developing colon cancer in the future.

Reduced Mortality: Regular screening has been shown to reduce the risk of dying from colon cancer. By detecting cancer at an early stage when it's most treatable or preventing it altogether, screening can help save lives.

Increased Survival Rates: Individuals whose colon cancer is detected at an early stage have higher survival rates compared to those whose cancer is diagnosed at a later stage. Screening allows for the detection of cancer at an earlier, more treatable stage, improving overall survival rates.

Improved Quality of Life: Early detection and treatment of colon cancer can help preserve quality of life by reducing the need for more aggressive treatments and minimizing the impact of the disease on daily functioning.

Cost-Effectiveness: While screening tests may incur initial costs, they are generally more cost-effective than treating advanced-stage colon cancer. By preventing cancer or detecting it early when treatment is less intensive, screening can help reduce healthcare costs in the long run.

Screening Tests

The choice of screening test depends on factors such as individual preferences, medical history, risk factors, and access to healthcare resources. It's essential to discuss screening options with a healthcare provider to determine the most appropriate test for each individual. Regular screening starting at age 45-50 for average-risk individuals can help detect colon cancer early and improve outcomes.

Colonoscopy: Colonoscopy is considered the gold standard for colon cancer screening. During this procedure, a flexible tube with a camera on the end (colonoscope) is inserted into the colon to examine the entire length of the colon and rectum. If polyps or abnormal tissue are found, they can be removed or biopsied during the procedure. Colonoscopy is recommended every 10 years for average-risk individuals starting at age 45-50.

Fecal Occult Blood Test (FOBT): FOBT is a non-invasive test that checks for the presence of blood in the stool, which can be a sign of colon cancer or precancerous polyps. This test can be done at home using a kit provided by a healthcare provider, and samples of stool are collected and sent to a laboratory for analysis. FOBT should be performed annually.

Fecal Immunochemical Test (FIT): Similar to FOBT, FIT is a stool-based test that checks for the presence of blood in the stool. FIT is more specific for human blood and may be preferred over FOBT. It also requires annual testing.

Stool DNA Test: Stool DNA tests, such as Cologuard, detect DNA changes associated with colon cancer and precancerous polyps in the stool. This test is also performed at home using a kit provided by a healthcare provider, and samples of stool are sent to a laboratory for analysis. Stool DNA tests are typically recommended every 3 years.

Flexible Sigmoidoscopy: Flexible sigmoidoscopy is a procedure that examines the lower part of the colon (sigmoid colon) and rectum using a flexible tube with a camera on the end (sigmoidoscope). While not as comprehensive as colonoscopy, sigmoidoscopy can detect most colon cancers and polyps in the lower part of the colon. It's typically recommended every 5 years, often in combination with FOBT or FIT.

CT Colonography (Virtual Colonoscopy): CT colonography is a non-invasive imaging test that uses computed tomography (CT) scans to create detailed images of the colon and rectum. It's less invasive than colonoscopy but still requires bowel preparation. If polyps or abnormalities are detected, a follow-up colonoscopy may be needed for further evaluation.

Screening Guidelines and Recommendations

Screening guidelines and recommendations for colon cancer vary slightly among different organizations, but there are general consensus guidelines based on age, risk factors, and individual preferences. Here are the common screening recommendations:

Average-Risk Individuals:

•**Age 45-50**: Screening for colon cancer is typically recommended to start at age 45-50 for average-risk individuals, regardless of gender.

•**Screening Intervals:** The preferred screening interval for most average-risk individuals is every 10 years, although some tests may be recommended more frequently.

High-Risk Individuals:

•**Family History:** Individuals with a family history of colon cancer or certain hereditary syndromes may need to start screening earlier and undergo more frequent screening. For example, those with a first-degree relative diagnosed with colon cancer before age 60 or two or more first-degree relatives diagnosed at any age may need to start screening at age 40 or 10 years before the age at which the youngest relative was diagnosed, whichever comes first.

•**Genetic Syndromes:** Individuals with known genetic syndromes such as familial adenomatous polyposis (FAP) or Lynch syndrome may require specialized screening protocols starting at a younger age.

Shared Decision-Making: It's important for individuals to discuss screening options with their healthcare provider to determine the most appropriate test based on their preferences, risk factors, and medical history. Shared decision-making allows for personalized screening recommendations that take into account individual preferences and values.

Follow-Up Testing: Individuals who have abnormal screening results or who are found to have polyps during screening may require follow-up testing or surveillance colonoscopies at shorter intervals to monitor for changes or recurrence.

It's essential to follow the screening guidelines recommended by healthcare providers and to undergo regular screening for colon cancer, as early detection can lead to better outcomes and a higher chance of cure.

Lifestyle Modifications for Prevention

Lifestyle modifications can play a significant role in reducing the risk of colon cancer. Here are some recommendations for preventing colon cancer through lifestyle changes:

Maintain a Healthy Weight: Aim to achieve and maintain a healthy weight through a balanced diet and regular physical activity. Obesity and being overweight are associated with an increased risk of colon cancer, so maintaining a healthy weight can help reduce your risk.

Eat a Healthy Diet: Focus on a diet rich in fruits, vegetables, whole grains, and lean proteins. Limit consumption of red and processed meats, as well as foods high in saturated fats and sugars. Include sources of fiber in your diet, such as beans, lentils, whole grains, fruits, and vegetables, which can help promote regular bowel movements and reduce the risk of colon cancer.

Limit Alcohol Consumption: Limit alcohol intake to moderate levels, which is defined as up to one drink per day for women and up to two drinks per day for men. Excessive alcohol consumption is associated with an increased risk of colon cancer.

Quit Smoking: If you smoke, quit smoking. Smoking is a known risk factor for several types of cancer, including colon cancer. Quitting smoking can reduce your risk of developing colon cancer and improve your overall health.

Be Physically Active: Engage in regular physical activity, such as brisk walking, jogging, cycling, swimming, or participating in sports. Aim for at least 150 minutes of moderate-intensity exercise or 75 minutes of vigorous-intensity exercise per week. Regular physical activity can help reduce the risk of colon cancer and improve overall health.

Screening: Follow recommended screening guidelines for colon cancer, starting at age 45-50 for average-risk individuals, or earlier if you have certain risk factors or a family history of colon cancer. Early detection through screening can help detect colon cancer in its early stages when it's most treatable.

Limit Processed Foods and Sugary Drinks: Limit consumption of processed foods, sugary snacks, and sugary beverages, as they are often high in unhealthy fats, sugars, and calories. Instead, opt for whole, unprocessed foods and choose water or other low-calorie beverages as your primary source of hydration.

Stay Hydrated: Drink plenty of water throughout the day to stay hydrated. Adequate hydration can help maintain healthy bowel function and reduce the risk of constipation, which is a risk factor for colon cancer.

By incorporating these lifestyle modifications into your daily routine, you can help reduce your risk of developing colon cancer and improve your overall health and well-being. It's essential to make sustainable lifestyle changes and maintain them over time for long-term health benefits.

Hereditary Syndromes and Screening Recommendations

Hereditary syndromes associated with an increased risk of colon cancer include familial adenomatous polyposis (FAP), Lynch syndrome (hereditary nonpolyposis colorectal cancer or HNPCC), and other less common syndromes. Here's an overview of these syndromes and their screening recommendations for colon cancer:

Familial Adenomatous Polyposis (FAP):

•**Description:** FAP is an inherited condition characterized by the development of hundreds to thousands of colorectal polyps in the colon and rectum, usually starting in the teenage years. Without treatment, individuals with FAP have a nearly 100% risk of developing colorectal cancer.

•**Screening Recommendations:** Screening for FAP typically involves genetic testing to identify mutations in the APC gene, which is responsible for the condition. Individuals with a known APC gene mutation or a family history of FAP may undergo regular colonoscopies starting in adolescence to detect and remove polyps before they become cancerous. Prophylactic colectomy (surgical removal of the colon) may be recommended in some cases to reduce the risk of colon cancer.

Lynch Syndrome (HNPCC):

•**Description:** Lynch syndrome is an inherited condition caused by mutations in genes responsible for DNA repair, such as MLH1, MSH2, MSH6, PMS2, and EPCAM. Individuals with Lynch syndrome have an increased risk of developing colorectal cancer, as well as other cancers including endometrial, ovarian, stomach, small intestine, pancreatic, and urinary tract cancers.

•**Screening Recommendations:** Screening for Lynch syndrome involves genetic testing to identify mutations in the associated genes. Individuals with Lynch syndrome may undergo more frequent colonoscopies starting at a younger age (often beginning in the late teens or early 20s) to detect and remove polyps before they become cancerous. Screening may also include regular surveillance for other associated cancers, such as endometrial cancer in women.

Other Hereditary Syndromes:

Other hereditary syndromes associated with an increased risk of colon cancer include MUTYH-associated polyposis (MAP), Peutz-Jeghers syndrome, juvenile polyposis syndrome, and Cowden syndrome, among others.

Screening Recommendations: Screening recommendations for these syndromes vary depending on the specific genetic mutation and associated cancer risks. Genetic counseling and testing are recommended for individuals with a personal or family history suggestive of hereditary colon cancer syndromes. Screening protocols may include colonoscopies, genetic testing, and surveillance for other associated cancers as appropriate.

It's essential for individuals with a family history of colon cancer or other risk factors to discuss screening recommendations with a healthcare provider or genetic counselor to determine the most appropriate screening protocol based on their individual circumstances. Early detection and appropriate surveillance can help reduce the risk of colon cancer and improve outcomes for individuals at increased risk due to hereditary syndromes.

Chapter 3: Treatment Options

Treatment Overview: Surgery, Chemotherapy, Radiation Therapy

Treatment for colon cancer often involves a combination of surgery, chemotherapy, and in some cases, radiation therapy. Here's an overview of each treatment modality:

Surgery:

•**Primary Treatment:** Surgery is the primary treatment for localized colon cancer, where the tumor is confined to the colon or rectum and has not spread to other parts of the body. The goal of surgery is to remove the tumor along with a portion of healthy tissue surrounding it (resection). In some cases, a segment of the colon or rectum may be removed (partial colectomy or anterior resection), while in others, the entire colon may need to be removed (total colectomy).

•**Lymph Node Dissection:** During surgery, nearby lymph nodes may also be removed and examined to determine if the cancer has spread beyond the primary tumor site.

•**Colostomy or Ileostomy:** In some cases, particularly when a significant portion of the colon or rectum is removed, a temporary or permanent colostomy or ileostomy may be necessary to divert stool from the remaining bowel to an opening in the abdominal wall.

Chemotherapy:

•**Adjuvant Therapy:** After surgery, some patients may receive adjuvant chemotherapy, which is chemotherapy given to kill any remaining cancer cells and reduce the risk of cancer recurrence. Adjuvant chemotherapy is typically recommended for patients with stage III colon cancer (cancer that has spread to nearby lymph nodes but not to distant organs).

•**Neoadjuvant Therapy:** In some cases, chemotherapy may be given before surgery (neoadjuvant chemotherapy) to shrink the tumor and make it easier to remove surgically. This approach is less common in colon cancer compared to other types of cancer.

Radiation Therapy:

Adjuvant or Neoadjuvant Therapy: Radiation therapy is less commonly used in the treatment of colon cancer compared to rectal cancer. It may be used in combination with chemotherapy (chemoradiation) as adjuvant or neoadjuvant therapy for rectal cancer to shrink the tumor and reduce the risk of recurrence. However, radiation therapy is not routinely used as part of the primary treatment for colon cancer.

Targeted Therapy and Immunotherapy:

•**Targeted Therapy:** Some patients with advanced or metastatic colon cancer may receive targeted therapy drugs, which specifically target cancer cells based on their genetic characteristics. Examples of targeted therapy drugs used in colon cancer treatment include cetuximab, panitumumab, bevacizumab, and regorafenib.

•**Immunotherapy:** Immunotherapy drugs, such as pembrolizumab and nivolumab, may also be used in some cases to boost the body's immune response against cancer cells. Immunotherapy is typically reserved for patients with certain genetic mutations or advanced-stage colon cancer that has not responded to other treatments.

The specific treatment approach for colon cancer depends on factors such as the stage of the cancer, the location of the tumor, the patient's overall health and preferences, and the presence of any genetic mutations or other factors that may affect treatment decisions. Treatment plans are developed by a multidisciplinary team of healthcare providers, including surgeons, medical oncologists, radiation oncologists, and other specialists, to provide the most comprehensive and personalized care for each patient.

Surgical Approaches: Colectomy, Laparoscopic Surgery, Robotic Surgery

Surgical approaches for the treatment of colon cancer typically involve removing the tumor along with a portion of healthy tissue surrounding it (resection). Several surgical techniques may be used, including traditional open colectomy, laparoscopic surgery, and robotic surgery. Here's an overview of each approach:

Open Colectomy:

•**Description:** Open colectomy is the traditional surgical approach for removing colon cancer. It involves making a large incision in the abdomen to access the colon and remove the tumor along with a portion of the surrounding healthy tissue.

•**Advantages**: Open colectomy allows the surgeon to have direct visualization and tactile feedback, which may be beneficial in certain cases, particularly for larger tumors or more complex surgeries.

•**Disadvantages:** Open colectomy requires a larger incision and longer recovery time compared to minimally invasive techniques. It may also be associated with increased postoperative pain and risk of complications.

Laparoscopic Surgery:

•**Description:** Laparoscopic surgery, also known as minimally invasive surgery, involves making several small incisions in the abdomen and inserting a laparoscope (a thin, flexible tube with a camera) and specialized surgical instruments to perform the procedure.

•**Advantages:** Laparoscopic surgery offers several advantages over open colectomy, including smaller incisions, less postoperative pain, shorter hospital stays, faster recovery times, and reduced risk of complications such as wound infections and hernias.

•**Disadvantages:** Laparoscopic surgery may not be suitable for all patients or all types of colon cancer, particularly in cases where the tumor is large or located in a difficult-to-reach area of the colon.

Robotic Surgery:

•**Description:** Robotic surgery is a type of minimally invasive surgery that uses robotic arms controlled by the surgeon to perform the procedure. Like laparoscopic surgery, robotic surgery involves making small incisions in the abdomen and inserting a camera and surgical instruments.

•**Advantages:** Robotic surgery offers several potential advantages over laparoscopic surgery, including enhanced dexterity and precision, improved visualization, and greater range of motion of the surgical instruments. This may be particularly beneficial for complex surgeries or in cases where the tumor is located in a challenging location.

•Disadvantages: Robotic surgery requires specialized equipment and training, which may not be available at all medical centers. It may also be associated with higher costs compared to traditional laparoscopic or open surgery.

The choice of surgical approach depends on factors such as the size and location of the tumor, the patient's overall health and preferences, and the expertise of the surgical team. It's essential for patients to discuss the pros and cons of each surgical approach with their healthcare provider to determine the most appropriate option for their individual circumstances.

Chemotherapy: Drugs, Side Effects, and Management

Chemotherapy is a systemic treatment for colon cancer that uses drugs to kill cancer cells or stop them from growing and dividing. Here's an overview of commonly used chemotherapy drugs for colon cancer, their side effects, and strategies for managing those side effects:

Chemotherapy Drugs:

•**5-Fluorouracil (5-FU):** 5-FU is one of the most commonly used chemotherapy drugs for colon cancer. It works by interfering with the synthesis of DNA and RNA in cancer cells, leading to cell death.

•**Capecitabine (Xeloda):** Capecitabine is an oral chemotherapy drug that is converted into 5-FU in the body. It is often used as an alternative to intravenous 5-FU for the treatment of colon cancer.

•**Oxaliplatin:** Oxaliplatin is a platinum-based chemotherapy drug that works by interfering with DNA replication and causing DNA damage in cancer cells.

•**Irinotecan:** Irinotecan is a topoisomerase inhibitor that works by blocking an enzyme called topoisomerase I, which is involved in DNA replication and repair.

•**Targeted Therapy:** In addition to traditional chemotherapy drugs, targeted therapy drugs such as cetuximab, panitumumab, bevacizumab, and regorafenib may be used in combination with chemotherapy to specifically target cancer cells based on their genetic characteristics.

Side Effects:

•**Nausea and Vomiting:** Chemotherapy drugs can cause nausea and vomiting, which can be managed with anti-nausea medications (antiemetics) prescribed by your healthcare provider.

•**Fatigue:** Chemotherapy can cause fatigue, which may persist throughout treatment. It's essential to get plenty of rest and conserve energy while undergoing chemotherapy.

•**Hair Loss:** Some chemotherapy drugs may cause hair loss, although not all patients experience this side effect. Hair loss is usually temporary, and hair typically grows back after treatment ends.

•**Low Blood Cell Counts:** Chemotherapy can suppress the bone marrow's ability to produce blood cells, leading to low white blood cell counts (neutropenia), low red blood cell counts (anemia), and low platelet counts (thrombocytopenia). This can increase the risk of infection, fatigue, and bleeding. Blood tests are often performed to monitor blood cell counts, and medications or blood transfusions may be given to manage low blood cell counts.

•**Peripheral Neuropathy:** Oxaliplatin and other chemotherapy drugs can cause peripheral neuropathy, a condition characterized by numbness, tingling, or pain in the hands and feet. Symptoms may improve after treatment ends, but in some cases, they may persist or worsen.

•**Diarrhea or Constipation:** Chemotherapy drugs can affect the digestive system, leading to diarrhea or constipation. It's essential to stay hydrated and follow dietary recommendations provided by your healthcare provider to manage these symptoms.

Management Strategies:

•**Medications:** Anti-nausea medications, pain relievers, and other supportive medications may be prescribed to manage chemotherapy side effects.

•**Dietary Changes:** Eating small, frequent meals and avoiding spicy, greasy, or heavy foods can help manage nausea and digestive symptoms. It's also essential to stay hydrated and maintain a balanced diet rich in fruits, vegetables, whole grains, and lean proteins.

•**Exercise:** Regular exercise can help combat fatigue and improve overall well-being during chemotherapy treatment. However, it's essential to consult with your healthcare provider before starting any exercise program.

•**Supportive Care:** Supportive care services such as counseling, support groups, and complementary therapies (e.g., acupuncture, massage) can provide emotional support and help manage treatment side effects.

It's essential to communicate openly with your healthcare provider about any side effects you experience during chemotherapy treatment. Your healthcare team can provide personalized recommendations and support to help manage side effects and optimize your treatment experience.

Radiation Therapy: Techniques and Side Effects

Radiation therapy, also known as radiotherapy, is a local treatment for colon cancer that uses high-energy X-rays or other types of radiation to kill cancer cells or stop them from growing and dividing. Here's an overview of radiation therapy techniques used for colon cancer and common side effects:

External Beam Radiation Therapy (EBRT):

•**Description:** EBRT is the most common type of radiation therapy used for colon cancer. It involves delivering radiation from a machine outside the body to the area of the colon or rectum where the tumor is located.

•**Technique:** During EBRT, the patient lies on a treatment table, and a machine called a linear accelerator delivers targeted radiation beams to the tumor site while sparing nearby healthy tissues as much as possible. The treatment is typically administered daily over several weeks.

•**Side Effects:** Common side effects of EBRT for colon cancer may include fatigue, skin irritation or redness in the treatment area, diarrhea, abdominal discomfort or cramping, and changes in bowel habits. These side effects are usually temporary and improve after treatment ends.

Brachytherapy:

•**Description:** Brachytherapy, also known as internal radiation therapy, involves placing radioactive sources directly into or near the tumor site.

•**Technique:** In the context of colon cancer, brachytherapy is less commonly used compared to EBRT. It may be used in select cases, such as for rectal cancer, where the radioactive sources are inserted into the rectum or surrounding tissues during surgery.

•**Side Effects:** Side effects of brachytherapy for colon cancer are similar to those of EBRT and may include fatigue, skin irritation, diarrhea, and changes in bowel habits.

Stereotactic Body Radiation Therapy (SBRT):

•Description: SBRT, also known as stereotactic ablative radiotherapy (SABR), is a highly precise form of radiation therapy that delivers high doses of radiation to the tumor in a small number of treatment sessions.

•Technique: SBRT uses advanced imaging techniques to precisely target the tumor while minimizing radiation exposure to surrounding healthy tissues. It may be used for localized colon cancers, particularly in cases where surgery is not an option.

•Side Effects: Side effects of SBRT for colon cancer may include fatigue, skin irritation, and gastrointestinal symptoms such as diarrhea or abdominal discomfort. These side effects are usually temporary and resolve after treatment.

Side Effects:

•Acute Side Effects: Common acute side effects of radiation therapy for colon cancer may include fatigue, skin irritation or redness in the treatment area, diarrhea, abdominal discomfort or cramping, and changes in bowel habits.

•Late Side Effects: Some patients may experience late side effects of radiation therapy months or years after treatment, including bowel or bladder problems, sexual dysfunction, and secondary cancers in the radiation field. However, these late side effects are rare, particularly with modern radiation techniques.

It's essential for patients undergoing radiation therapy for colon cancer to communicate openly with their healthcare providers about any side effects they experience during treatment. Your healthcare team can provide supportive care and recommend strategies to manage side effects and optimize your treatment experience.

Targeted Therapy and Immunotherapy

Targeted therapy and immunotherapy are newer treatment approaches for colon cancer that specifically target cancer cells or boost the body's immune response against cancer. Here's an overview of targeted therapy and immunotherapy for colon cancer:

Targeted Therapy:

•**Description:** Targeted therapy drugs are designed to interfere with specific molecules or pathways involved in the growth and spread of cancer cells. By targeting these specific molecules or pathways, targeted therapy drugs can block the growth of cancer cells while sparing normal cells.

•**Common Targeted Therapy Drugs:** Several targeted therapy drugs are approved for the treatment of advanced or metastatic colon cancer, including:

•**Cetuximab (Erbitux) and panitumumab (Vectibix):** These drugs target the epidermal growth factor receptor (EGFR), which is often overexpressed in colon cancer cells. They are used in combination with chemotherapy for certain patients with metastatic colon cancer.

•**Bevacizumab (Avastin):** Bevacizumab is a monoclonal antibody that targets vascular endothelial growth factor (VEGF), a protein that stimulates the growth of blood vessels. It is used in combination with chemotherapy for certain patients with metastatic colon cancer.

Immunotherapy:

•**Description:** Immunotherapy, also known as biologic therapy, harnesses the power of the body's immune system to recognize and attack cancer cells. Immunotherapy drugs work by stimulating the immune system or blocking inhibitory signals that prevent the immune system from recognizing and attacking cancer cells.

•**Common Immunotherapy Drugs:** While immunotherapy is not yet widely used for the treatment of colon cancer compared to other cancers, several immunotherapy drugs are being studied in clinical trials for colon cancer, including:

•**Pembrolizumab (Keytruda) and nivolumab (Opdivo):** These drugs are immune checkpoint inhibitors that target proteins such as programmed cell death protein 1 (PD-1) or programmed death-ligand 1 (PD-L1), which are involved in suppressing the immune response. They have shown promising results in clinical trials for patients with advanced or metastatic colon cancer who have certain genetic mutations or microsatellite instability-high (MSI-H) tumors.

Combination Therapy: Targeted therapy and immunotherapy may be used alone or in combination with chemotherapy or other treatments for colon cancer, depending on the specific characteristics of the tumor and the patient's overall health and preferences.

Side Effects: While targeted therapy and immunotherapy drugs are generally well tolerated, they can cause side effects similar to those of chemotherapy, including fatigue, nausea, diarrhea, skin rash, and immune-related adverse events such as inflammation of the lungs, liver, or intestines. It's essential for patients receiving targeted therapy or immunotherapy to communicate openly with their healthcare providers about any side effects they experience during treatment.

Personalized Medicine: Targeted therapy and immunotherapy drugs are part of a broader trend towards personalized medicine, where treatments are tailored to the specific characteristics of the individual patient and their tumor. Genetic testing and other molecular profiling techniques can help identify patients who are most likely to benefit from targeted therapy or immunotherapy.

Overall, targeted therapy and immunotherapy have transformed the treatment landscape for colon cancer, offering new options for patients with advanced or metastatic disease and improving outcomes for many patients. Ongoing research continues to explore new targeted therapy and immunotherapy drugs and combination treatment approaches for colon cancer.

Clinical Trials and Experimental Treatments

Clinical Trials test new treatments, treatment combinations, and approaches to improve outcomes for patients. Here's an overview of clinical trials and experimental treatments for colon cancer:

Clinical Trials:

•**Description:** Clinical trials are research studies that evaluate the safety and efficacy of new drugs, treatment strategies, or medical devices in human subjects. They are conducted to answer specific scientific questions and to gather evidence to support the approval of new treatments by regulatory authorities.

•**Phases of Clinical Trials:**

•**Phase I:** Phase I trials test the safety and dosing of a new treatment in a small group of patients to determine the maximum tolerated dose and potential side effects.

•**Phase II:** Phase II trials evaluate the effectiveness of a new treatment in a larger group of patients to further assess safety and efficacy.

•**Phase III:** Phase III trials compare the new treatment to standard treatments or placebo in a larger group of patients to determine if it is more effective, safer, or both.

•**Phase IV:** Phase IV trials, also known as post-marketing surveillance trials, are conducted after a treatment has been approved and are designed to monitor its long-term safety and effectiveness in real-world settings.

•**Benefits of Clinical Trials:** Participating in a clinical trial may offer access to new treatments not available outside of the trial, as well as the opportunity to contribute to medical research and help advance the understanding of colon cancer.

Experimental Treatments:

•**Description:** Experimental treatments are new therapies or treatment approaches that are being studied in preclinical or clinical research settings. They may include targeted therapy drugs, immunotherapy drugs, novel chemotherapy regimens, or innovative treatment strategies such as gene therapy or personalized medicine approaches.

•**Examples of Experimental Treatments:** Some examples of experimental treatments being studied for colon cancer include:

•Novel targeted therapy drugs that target specific genetic mutations or signaling pathways in colon cancer cells.

•Immunotherapy drugs that enhance the body's immune response against colon cancer.

•Combination treatment approaches that combine targeted therapy, immunotherapy, and chemotherapy to improve outcomes for patients.

•Innovative surgical techniques, radiation therapy approaches, or interventional radiology procedures.

•**Risks and Considerations:** Experimental treatments may carry unknown risks, and their safety and effectiveness have not been fully established. Patients considering participation in a clinical trial should discuss the potential risks and benefits with their healthcare provider and carefully weigh their options.

Finding Clinical Trials:

•Patients interested in participating in a clinical trial can search for trials relevant to colon cancer using online databases such as ClinicalTrials.gov, which is maintained by the National Institutes of Health (NIH). Healthcare providers can also help patients find appropriate clinical trials and provide information about eligibility criteria and enrollment processes.

Informed Consent:

•Before participating in a clinical trial, patients are required to provide informed consent, which involves understanding the purpose of the trial, the potential risks and benefits, and their rights as participants. Patients should ask questions and carefully review all relevant information before consenting to participate in a clinical trial.

Overall, clinical trials and experimental treatments offer hope for improving outcomes and advancing the treatment of colon cancer. Participation in clinical trials is voluntary and requires careful consideration of the potential risks and benefits, but it can provide access to promising new treatments and contribute to the advancement of medical knowledge.

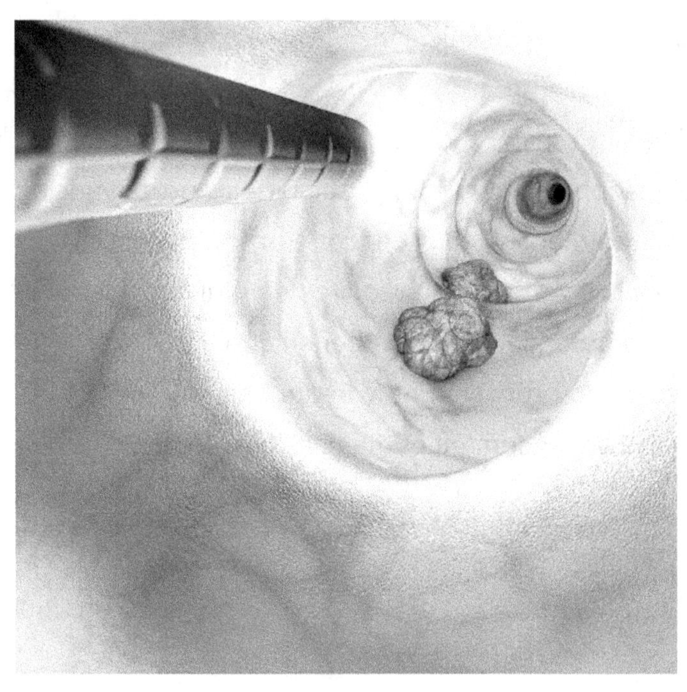

Chapter 4: Living with Colorectal Cancer

Coping with Diagnosis and Treatment

Being diagnosed with colon cancer and undergoing treatment can be a challenging and emotional experience. Here are some strategies for coping with the diagnosis and treatment of colon cancer:

Seek Support: Reach out to friends, family members, or support groups for emotional support. Talking to others who have gone through a similar experience can provide reassurance, encouragement, and practical advice.

Educate Yourself: Learn as much as you can about colon cancer, including the treatment options available, potential side effects, and self-care strategies. Knowledge can help you feel more empowered and in control of your treatment journey.

Communicate with Your Healthcare Team: Maintain open and honest communication with your healthcare providers about your concerns, questions, and treatment preferences. Your healthcare team can provide information, guidance, and support throughout the treatment process.

Take Care of Your Emotional Well-Being: Practice self-care activities such as meditation, deep breathing exercises, yoga, or mindfulness to reduce stress and promote emotional well-being. Consider seeking professional counseling or therapy if you're struggling to cope with the emotional impact of the diagnosis and treatment.

Stay Active: Engage in regular physical activity, such as walking, swimming, or gentle exercises, to help maintain your strength, energy levels, and overall well-being during treatment. Consult with your healthcare provider before starting any new exercise program.

Maintain a Healthy Diet: Eat a balanced diet rich in fruits, vegetables, whole grains, and lean proteins to support your immune system and overall health during treatment. Avoid foods that may aggravate digestive symptoms or interfere with treatment, and stay hydrated by drinking plenty of water.

Manage Side Effects: Work with your healthcare team to manage any side effects of treatment, such as nausea, fatigue, or pain. They can recommend medications, lifestyle changes, or supportive care strategies to help alleviate symptoms and improve your quality of life.

Stay Connected: Stay connected with your loved ones, friends, and support network throughout your treatment journey. Sharing your experiences, concerns, and victories with others can provide emotional support and help you feel less isolated.

Set Realistic Expectations: Understand that the treatment process may have ups and downs, and it's normal to experience a range of emotions throughout your journey. Set realistic expectations for yourself and be patient with yourself as you navigate the challenges of diagnosis and treatment.

Celebrate Milestones: Celebrate milestones and achievements, no matter how small, during your treatment journey. Whether it's completing a round of chemotherapy, reaching a treatment goal, or experiencing a day with reduced symptoms, take time to acknowledge and celebrate your progress.

Remember that coping with colon cancer is a personal journey, and it's okay to seek support and assistance along the way. Be kind to yourself, prioritize self-care, and lean on your support network for strength and encouragement during this challenging time.

Nutritional Guidance During Treatment

Nutritional guidance during colon cancer treatment is essential to help maintain strength, energy levels, and overall well-being while managing treatment side effects.

Daily dietary choices for colorectal cancer prevention;

The food and drinks you consume can be powerful tools for colorectal cancer prevention. A nutritious regular diet can improve your gut health, which is a main contributor to colon and rectal health.

Think of food as medicine-when you're mindful about the products you're consuming, you can arm your body with the nutrients it needs to prevent or fight off cancer cells.

Healthy practices to reduce risks and prevent colorectal cancer

Smart food choices can reduce the risk of colorectal cancer. In general, the American Cancer Society recommends that adults and children choose diets rich in high-fiber foods, such as whole fruits, veggies and whole grains. Practices for prevention include:

• **Increasing your dietary fiber intake.**

Consume fiber-rich foods, such as whole wheat bread or brown rice, beans and legumes,Lentils, peas.

What to choose:

• **Whole grains.** Brown rice, oats, 100% whole wheat bread products, quinoa, faro, barley and whole grain pasta.

• **Dairy products.** Low-fat milk, yogurt, cottage cheese and other cheese products.

Cancer research suggests the high calcium content in these may be protective.

• **Non-starchy vegetables and raw fruits.**

These are high in fiber, which promotes gut health. These also contain phytonutrients known to prevent many types of cancer.

What to lose:

• **Alcohol**. If you do drink alcohol, try to do so only occasionally and limit to two standard drinks per day for men or one standard drink per day for women

• **Red and processed meats.** Processed meat is any meat (white or dark) that has been preserved through salting, smoking or curing (such as salami, sausage, bologna, lunch meats and hot dogs). Both red meat and processed meat contain compounds that increase the risk of colon cancer.

Oatmeal, quinoa, whole-grain bread, and cereals are all great choices for breakfast. Whole grains are a good source of dietary fiber, magnesium and plant polyphenol compounds.

There is strong scientific evidence that eating whole grains decreases the risk of colorectal cancer.

Try to eat at least 3-5 servings of non-starchy vegetables per day, including lettuce, kale, cucumbers, artichokes, broccoli, cabbage, carrots, cauliflower, celery, okra and spinach. Protein is crucial for muscle development, growth of tissues and more.

Here are some dietary recommendations to consider during treatment:

Eat a Balanced Diet: Focus on consuming a balanced diet that includes a variety of nutrient-rich foods from all food groups. This includes fruits, vegetables, whole grains, lean proteins, and healthy fats.

Stay Hydrated: Drink plenty of fluids throughout the day to stay hydrated. Aim for at least 8-10 cups of water daily, and include hydrating beverages such as herbal teas, clear broths, and diluted fruit juices.

Include Protein-Rich Foods: Protein is essential for maintaining muscle mass and supporting the immune system during treatment. Include protein-rich foods such as lean meats, poultry, fish, eggs, dairy products, legumes, nuts, and seeds in your diet.

Consume Fiber-Rich Foods: Fiber can help promote regular bowel movements and prevent constipation, which may be a side effect of certain treatments. Choose fiber-rich foods such as fruits, vegetables, whole grains, beans, lentils, and nuts.

Manage Digestive Symptoms: If you experience digestive symptoms such as nausea, vomiting, diarrhea, or constipation, modify your diet to help alleviate discomfort. Eat small, frequent meals and avoid spicy, greasy, or heavy foods that may aggravate symptoms. Consider working with a registered dietitian who can provide personalized dietary recommendations based on your individual needs and preferences.

Opt for Easy-to-Digest Foods: During periods of treatment-related nausea or digestive discomfort, choose easy-to-digest foods such as plain crackers, toast, bananas, rice, applesauce, boiled potatoes, steamed vegetables, and broth-based soups.

Stay Mindful of Food Safety: Pay attention to food safety practices to reduce the risk of foodborne illness, which can be particularly important during treatment when the immune system may be compromised. Wash fruits and vegetables thoroughly, cook meats and eggs thoroughly, and avoid unpasteurized dairy products, raw seafood, and other high-risk foods.

Consider Nutritional Supplements: In some cases, nutritional supplements such as protein shakes, meal replacement drinks, or oral nutritional supplements may be recommended to help meet your nutritional needs during treatment. Talk to your healthcare provider or registered dietitian about whether supplements are appropriate for you.

Listen to Your Body: Listen to your body's cues and eat according to your appetite and tolerance level. If you're struggling to eat or experiencing significant weight loss during treatment, talk to your healthcare provider or dietitian for additional support and guidance.

Maintain Overall Health: In addition to dietary considerations, prioritize overall health by getting plenty of rest, engaging in regular physical activity as tolerated, and managing stress through relaxation techniques such as deep breathing, meditation, or yoga.

Remember that nutritional needs may vary depending on individual factors such as treatment regimen, treatment side effects, and overall health status. It's essential to work closely with your healthcare team and registered dietitian to develop a personalized nutrition plan that meets your individual needs and supports your overall health and well-being during colon cancer treatment.

Managing Side Effects: Fatigue, Nausea, Diarrhea, Neuropathy

Managing side effects during colon cancer treatment is crucial for maintaining quality of life and overall well-being. Here are some strategies for managing common side effects such as fatigue, nausea, diarrhea, and neuropathy:

Fatigue:

•**Get Adequate Rest:** Prioritize rest and sleep to help combat fatigue. Aim for 7-9 hours of quality sleep per night, and take short naps or breaks throughout the day as needed.

•**Stay Active:** Engage in gentle physical activity such as walking, yoga, or tai chi to help boost energy levels and reduce fatigue. Start with low-intensity exercises and gradually increase activity levels as tolerated.

•**Conserve Energy:** Pace yourself and conserve energy by prioritizing tasks, delegating responsibilities, and taking breaks when needed. Listen to your body and avoid overexertion.

Nausea:

•**Eat Small, Frequent Meals**: Instead of large meals, eat small, frequent meals throughout the day to help prevent nausea and maintain blood sugar levels. Choose bland, easily digestible foods such as crackers, toast, rice, bananas, and applesauce.

•**Stay Hydrated:** Sip on clear fluids such as water, herbal tea, ginger ale, or diluted fruit juice to stay hydrated and alleviate nausea. Avoid drinking large amounts of fluids with meals, as this can worsen nausea.

•**Use Anti-Nausea Medications:** Take anti-nausea medications (antiemetics) as prescribed by your healthcare provider to help alleviate nausea and vomiting. Be sure to follow the dosing instructions carefully and report any persistent or severe symptoms to your healthcare team.

Diarrhea:

•**Stay Hydrated:** Drink plenty of fluids to stay hydrated and replace lost electrolytes. Opt for clear fluids such as water, broth, sports drinks, and oral rehydration solutions to help prevent dehydration.

•**Follow a Low-Fiber Diet:** During episodes of diarrhea, follow a low-fiber diet that includes easily digestible foods such as bananas, rice, applesauce, toast, boiled potatoes, and well-cooked vegetables. Avoid high-fiber foods, spicy foods, caffeine, and dairy products, which can exacerbate diarrhea.

•**Consider Anti-Diarrheal Medications:** Talk to your healthcare provider about using over-the-counter or prescription anti-diarrheal medications such as loperamide (Imodium) to help control diarrhea. Be sure to follow the dosing instructions provided by your healthcare provider.

Neuropathy:

•**Manage Pain:** If neuropathy causes pain or discomfort, talk to your healthcare provider about pain management strategies such as over-the-counter or prescription pain medications, topical treatments, or nerve pain medications.

•**Protect Hands and Feet:** Take precautions to protect your hands and feet from injury and minimize further damage to nerves. Wear gloves when handling hot or cold objects, use padded insoles or cushioned shoes to reduce pressure on the feet, and avoid tight-fitting shoes or socks that may exacerbate symptoms.

•**Maintain Good Foot Care:** Practice good foot care habits such as inspecting your feet daily for cuts, sores, or blisters, keeping your feet clean and dry, and moisturizing your skin regularly to prevent dryness and cracking.

•**Consider Physical Therapy:** Physical therapy or occupational therapy may be beneficial for managing neuropathy-related symptoms and improving mobility and function. These therapies may include exercises, stretches, and techniques to improve strength, flexibility, and balance.

It's essential to communicate openly with your healthcare provider about any side effects you experience during colon cancer treatment. Your healthcare team can provide personalized recommendations and support to help manage side effects and improve your quality of life during treatment.

Emotional and Psychological Support

Emotional and psychological support is crucial for individuals facing a diagnosis of colon cancer and undergoing treatment. Here are some strategies for finding support and managing the emotional impact of colon cancer:

Talk to Your Healthcare Team: Your healthcare team can provide information, support, and resources to help you cope with the emotional challenges of colon cancer. Don't hesitate to discuss your feelings, concerns, and questions with your doctors, nurses, social workers, or other members of your healthcare team.

Seek Support from Loved Ones: Lean on friends, family members, and loved ones for emotional support during this challenging time. Share your feelings and concerns with those you trust, and allow them to provide comfort, encouragement, and practical assistance as needed.

Join a Support Group: Consider joining a support group for individuals with colon cancer or cancer survivors. Support groups provide a safe and supportive environment to share experiences, exchange advice, and connect with others who understand what you're going through. You can find local support groups through hospitals, cancer centers, or community organizations, or join online support groups and forums.

Consider Counseling or Therapy: Professional counseling or therapy can be beneficial for individuals struggling to cope with the emotional impact of colon cancer. A licensed therapist or counselor can provide individual or group therapy sessions to help you process your feelings, develop coping strategies, and navigate the challenges of diagnosis and treatment.

Practice Self-Care: Take time for self-care activities that promote relaxation, stress reduction, and emotional well-being. Engage in activities such as meditation, deep breathing exercises, mindfulness, yoga, journaling, or spending time in nature. Prioritize activities that bring you joy, fulfillment, and a sense of peace.

Stay Informed: Educate yourself about colon cancer, treatment options, and self-care strategies to empower yourself and reduce anxiety and uncertainty. Knowledge can help you feel more prepared and in control of your treatment journey.

Express Your Feelings: Allow yourself to express a range of emotions, including fear, sadness, anger, or frustration, in a healthy and constructive way. Talk to someone you trust, write in a journal, or engage in creative outlets such as art, music, or poetry to express your feelings and emotions.

Stay Connected: Stay connected with your support network, community, or spiritual/religious community for emotional and spiritual support. Share your journey with others, participate in meaningful activities, and draw strength from your connections and relationships.

Set Realistic Expectations: Be kind to yourself and set realistic expectations for coping with the emotional challenges of colon cancer. Understand that it's normal to experience a range of emotions during this time, and give yourself permission to take things one day at a time.

Seek Professional Help if Needed: If you're struggling to cope with the emotional impact of colon cancer or experiencing symptoms of depression, anxiety, or distress, don't hesitate to seek professional help. Talk to your healthcare provider or mental health professional about your feelings and concerns, and explore options for counseling, therapy, or medication as appropriate.

Remember that coping with colon cancer is a personal journey, and it's okay to seek support and assistance along the way. Take care of yourself, prioritize your emotional well-being, and reach out for help when needed.

Integrative Therapies: Acupuncture, Massage, Yoga

Integrative therapies such as acupuncture, massage, and yoga can complement traditional medical treatments for colon cancer by promoting relaxation, reducing stress, alleviating treatment side effects, and improving overall well-being. Here's how each of these integrative therapies can be beneficial:

Acupuncture:

•**Description:** Acupuncture is a traditional Chinese medicine technique that involves the insertion of thin needles into specific points on the body to stimulate energy flow and promote healing. It is believed to help restore balance to the body's energy (qi) and relieve pain and other symptoms.

•**Benefits:** Acupuncture may help alleviate treatment-related side effects such as nausea, vomiting, fatigue, pain, neuropathy, and anxiety. It can also promote relaxation, improve sleep quality, and enhance overall well-being.

•**Safety:** Acupuncture is generally considered safe when performed by a licensed and trained practitioner using sterile needles. However, it's essential to consult with your healthcare provider before starting acupuncture, especially if you have a compromised immune system or are taking blood-thinning medications.

Massage Therapy:

•**Description:** Massage therapy involves the manipulation of soft tissues (muscles, tendons, ligaments) to promote relaxation, reduce muscle tension, and alleviate pain. Different massage techniques, such as Swedish massage, deep tissue massage, and aromatherapy massage, may be used depending on individual preferences and needs.

•**Benefits:** Massage therapy can help reduce stress, anxiety, and depression, improve circulation, enhance lymphatic drainage, and relieve muscle tension and pain. It may also help alleviate treatment-related side effects such as fatigue, neuropathy, and digestive issues.

•**Safety:** Massage therapy is generally safe for most people, but it's essential to communicate openly with your massage therapist about your medical history, treatment regimen, and any areas of concern. Choose a licensed and experienced massage therapist who is familiar with working with cancer patients.

Yoga:

•**Description:** Yoga is a mind-body practice that combines physical postures, breathwork, meditation, and relaxation techniques to promote balance, flexibility, strength, and inner peace. Various styles of yoga, such as Hatha yoga, Vinyasa yoga, and Restorative yoga, may be suitable for individuals with cancer.

•**Benefits:** Yoga can help reduce stress, anxiety, and depression, improve sleep quality, increase flexibility and strength, and enhance overall well-being. It may also help alleviate treatment-related side effects such as fatigue, neuropathy, and digestive issues.

•**Safety:** Yoga is generally safe for most people, but it's essential to choose appropriate yoga poses and modifications based on individual abilities and limitations. Inform your yoga instructor about your medical history, treatment regimen, and any physical limitations or concerns.

Before starting any integrative therapy, it's essential to consult with your healthcare provider to ensure that it is safe and appropriate for your individual circumstances. Integrative therapies should complement, not replace, traditional medical treatments for colon cancer. Additionally, choose qualified and experienced practitioners who have expertise in working with individuals with cancer.

Sexual Health and Fertility Concerns

Sexual health and fertility concerns are important aspects of the cancer journey, including colon cancer. Here are some considerations and strategies for addressing sexual health and fertility concerns during and after colon cancer treatment:

Open Communication: It's essential to communicate openly with your healthcare team about any sexual health or fertility concerns you may have. Your healthcare providers can provide information, guidance, and support tailored to your individual needs and circumstances.

Understand Treatment Effects: Some treatments for colon cancer, such as surgery, chemotherapy, and radiation therapy, can have temporary or long-term effects on sexual function and fertility. Surgery to remove part of the colon or rectum may affect bowel function, which can impact sexual activity. Chemotherapy and radiation therapy can also affect hormone levels, fertility, and sexual function.

Address Physical Symptoms: If you experience physical symptoms such as fatigue, pain, nausea, or bowel changes that impact your sexual health or fertility, talk to your healthcare provider about managing these symptoms. Addressing physical symptoms can help improve overall well-being and quality of life.

Explore Sexual Health Resources: Many cancer centers and healthcare facilities offer sexual health resources and support services for individuals with cancer. These resources may include counseling, education, support groups, and referrals to sexual health specialists or therapists who can address sexual health concerns.

Consider Fertility Preservation: If fertility preservation is a concern, discuss your options with your healthcare provider before starting cancer treatment. Depending on individual circumstances, options for fertility preservation may include sperm banking for men, egg or embryo freezing for women, or other assisted reproductive technologies.

Adapt and Experiment: Experiment with different sexual positions, techniques, or intimacy practices that are comfortable and enjoyable for you and your partner. Be patient and open-minded, and focus on connecting emotionally and physically with your partner.

Address Emotional and Psychological Factors: Coping with a cancer diagnosis and undergoing treatment can have emotional and psychological effects that impact sexual health and intimacy. Seek support from a counselor, therapist, or support group to address emotional and psychological concerns and strengthen coping skills.

Take Care of Overall Health: Taking care of your overall health and well-being can positively impact sexual health and fertility. Eat a balanced diet, engage in regular physical activity, manage stress, prioritize sleep, and avoid tobacco, alcohol, and recreational drugs.

Involve Your Partner: Include your partner in discussions about sexual health and fertility concerns, and work together as a team to address challenges and find solutions. Open communication and mutual support are essential for maintaining intimacy and connection during the cancer journey.

Be Patient and Gentle with Yourself: Remember that sexual health and fertility concerns are common and normal aspects of the cancer experience. Be patient and gentle with yourself, and give yourself permission to explore, adapt, and adjust as needed.

Overall, addressing sexual health and fertility concerns requires open communication, support from healthcare providers, and a willingness to explore and adapt to changes. By addressing these concerns proactively and seeking appropriate support, individuals with colon cancer can maintain intimacy, connection, and overall well-being throughout the treatment journey and beyond.

Support for Caregivers and Loved Ones

Support for caregivers and loved ones of individuals with colon cancer is crucial for providing emotional support, practical assistance, and maintaining their own well-being during the cancer journey. Here are some strategies and resources for supporting caregivers and loved ones:

Educate Yourself: Learn as much as you can about colon cancer, treatment options, and potential side effects to better understand what your loved one is going through. Knowledge can help caregivers feel more empowered and prepared to provide support.

Seek Support from Others: Caregivers should not hesitate to seek support from friends, family members, support groups, or professional counselors. Sharing experiences and connecting with others who understand can provide emotional validation, encouragement, and practical advice.

Take Care of Yourself: Caregivers often neglect their own needs while focusing on the needs of their loved ones. It's essential for caregivers to prioritize self-care activities such as getting enough rest, eating a healthy diet, engaging in physical activity, and seeking respite when needed.

Set Boundaries: Establish clear boundaries and realistic expectations for caregiving responsibilities. Communicate openly with your loved one about what you can and cannot do, and don't hesitate to ask for help or delegate tasks to other family members or friends.

Respect Autonomy: Respect your loved one's autonomy and decisions regarding their treatment and care. Offer support and assistance without trying to control or dictate their choices.

Offer Practical Support: Provide practical assistance with daily tasks such as meal preparation, transportation to medical appointments, managing medications, and household chores. Even small gestures of support can make a significant difference to someone undergoing cancer treatment.

Be Flexible and Adaptive: Understand that caregiving responsibilities may change over time as treatment progresses and circumstances evolve. Be flexible and adaptive in your approach to caregiving, and be willing to adjust plans and expectations as needed.

Acknowledge Your Feelings: Caregiving can evoke a wide range of emotions, including stress, sadness, frustration, guilt, and even resentment. Acknowledge and validate your feelings, and seek support from others to help you cope with the emotional challenges of caregiving.

Access Resources and Support Services: Take advantage of resources and support services available to caregivers, such as respite care, support groups, counseling services, and educational programs. Many cancer centers and healthcare facilities offer support services specifically designed for caregivers.

Remember that caregiving is a journey that requires patience, compassion, and resilience. By taking care of yourself and seeking support from others, you can better support your loved one with colon cancer while maintaining your own well-being

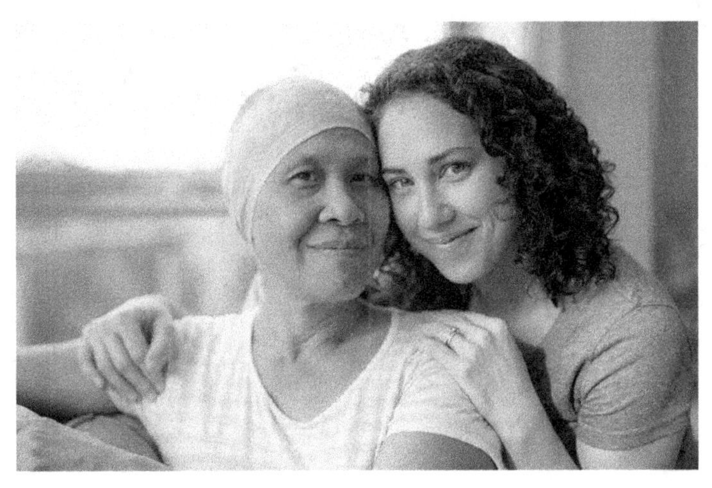

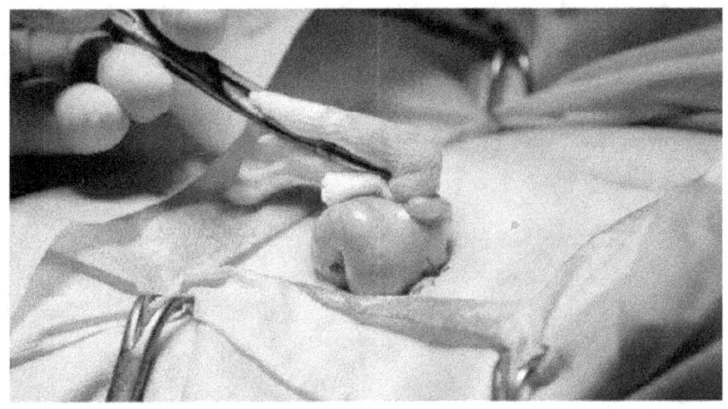

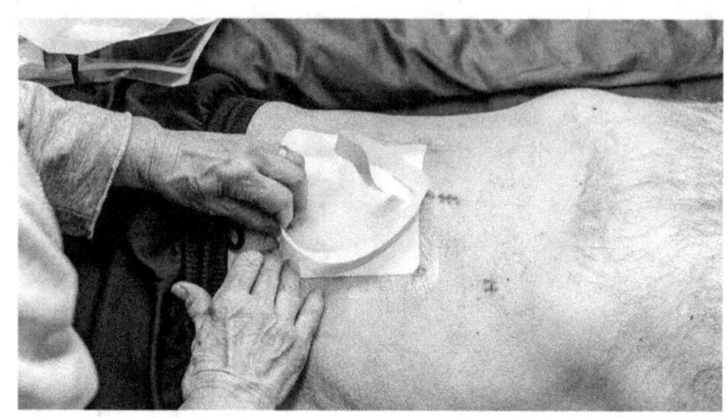

Chapter 5: Survivorship and Beyond

Life After Treatment: Follow-Up Care and Surveillance

Life after colon cancer treatment involves ongoing follow-up care and surveillance to monitor for recurrence, manage potential long-term side effects, and promote overall health and well-being. Here are some key aspects of follow-up care and surveillance for individuals who have completed treatment for colon cancer:

Follow-Up Appointments: Attend regular follow-up appointments with your healthcare provider, typically every three to six months in the first few years after treatment, and then less frequently over time. These appointments may include physical exams, blood tests, imaging studies (such as CT scans or colonoscopies), and other tests to monitor for signs of recurrence or complications.

Colonoscopy: Colonoscopies are typically recommended as part of surveillance for colon cancer survivors. The timing and frequency of colonoscopies will depend on individual factors such as the stage of the cancer, the type of treatment received, and the presence of any pre-cancerous polyps. Your healthcare provider will provide guidance on when to schedule your next colonoscopy.

Imaging Studies: In addition to colonoscopies, your healthcare provider may recommend periodic imaging studies such as CT scans, MRI scans, or PET scans to monitor for recurrence or metastasis of colon cancer. The frequency and type of imaging studies will depend on your individual risk factors and treatment history.

Blood Tests: Routine blood tests, including tests to monitor tumor markers such as carcinoembryonic antigen (CEA), may be performed during follow-up appointments to help detect signs of recurrence or monitor treatment response.

Symptom Monitoring: Be vigilant about monitoring for any new or recurring symptoms that could indicate a recurrence of colon cancer, such as unexplained weight loss, abdominal pain, changes in bowel habits, blood in the stool, or persistent fatigue. Report any concerning symptoms to your healthcare provider promptly.

Healthy Lifestyle: Maintain a healthy lifestyle to reduce the risk of cancer recurrence and promote overall health and well-being. This includes eating a balanced diet, engaging in regular physical activity, maintaining a healthy weight, avoiding tobacco and excessive alcohol consumption, and managing stress.

Psychosocial Support: Life after cancer treatment can bring a range of emotions, including fear, anxiety, and uncertainty. Seek support from friends, family members, support groups, or mental health professionals to address emotional and psychological concerns and cope with the transition to survivorship.

Long-Term Side Effect Management: Some individuals may experience long-term side effects of colon cancer treatment, such as bowel dysfunction, neuropathy, fatigue, or emotional distress. Work with your healthcare provider to manage these side effects and address any ongoing concerns or challenges.

Genetic Counseling and Testing: For individuals with a family history of colon cancer or a known genetic predisposition to the disease, genetic counseling and testing may be recommended to assess the risk of recurrence or the development of other cancers. Discuss these options with your healthcare provider if applicable.

Stay Informed: Stay informed about advances in colon cancer research, treatment options, and survivorship care. Participate in survivorship programs, educational workshops, or online resources to stay up-to-date and empowered in managing your post-treatment care.

Life after colon cancer treatment is a journey that requires ongoing vigilance, self-care, and support. By staying engaged in follow-up care and surveillance, maintaining a healthy lifestyle, and seeking support as needed, individuals can optimize their health and well-being as they transition to survivorship.

Survivorship Care Plans

Survivorship care plans are personalized documents that provide cancer survivors with important information and guidance to help them navigate life after cancer treatment. These plans typically include a summary of the individual's cancer diagnosis, treatment history, and recommendations for follow-up care and surveillance. Here are the key components of survivorship care plans for individuals who have completed treatment for colon cancer:

Patient Information: The survivorship care plan begins with basic demographic information about the individual, including their name, date of birth, contact information, and any relevant medical history.

Cancer Diagnosis and Treatment Summary: This section provides a summary of the individual's colon cancer diagnosis, including the cancer stage, tumor characteristics, and any relevant pathology findings. It also outlines the treatments received, including surgery, chemotherapy, radiation therapy, and any other interventions.

Follow-Up Care Recommendations: The survivorship care plan includes specific recommendations for follow-up care and surveillance based on the individual's cancer diagnosis, treatment history, and risk factors. This may include recommendations for regular physical exams, blood tests, imaging studies (such as colonoscopies or CT scans), and other tests to monitor for signs of recurrence or complications.

Long-Term Side Effect Management: This section addresses potential long-term side effects of colon cancer treatment and provides guidance on managing these side effects. It may include recommendations for managing bowel dysfunction, neuropathy, fatigue, emotional distress, and other common issues experienced by cancer survivors.

Healthy Lifestyle Recommendations: Survivorship care plans often include recommendations for maintaining a healthy lifestyle to reduce the risk of cancer recurrence and promote overall health and well-being. This may include guidance on diet, exercise, weight management, tobacco cessation, and alcohol moderation.

Psychosocial Support Resources: Recognizing the emotional and psychological challenges faced by cancer survivors, survivorship care plans may include information about psychosocial support resources such as support groups, counseling services, online communities, and educational programs.

Genetic Counseling and Testing: For individuals with a family history of colon cancer or a known genetic predisposition to the disease, survivorship care plans may include recommendations for genetic counseling and testing to assess the risk of recurrence or the development of other cancers.

Healthcare Provider Contacts: The survivorship care plan typically includes contact information for the individual's healthcare providers, including primary care physicians, oncologists, specialists, and other members of the healthcare team involved in their care.

Personalized Recommendations: Survivorship care plans are personalized to the individual's unique needs, preferences, and circumstances. Recommendations may be tailored based on factors such as age, sex, comorbidities, treatment history, and risk factors.

Follow-Up Schedule: Finally, survivorship care plans often include a schedule for follow-up appointments and tests, outlining when and how often the individual should be seen by their healthcare providers for ongoing monitoring and surveillance.

Survivorship care plans serve as valuable tools to empower cancer survivors with information, resources, and support as they transition from active treatment to survivorship. They help individuals understand their cancer journey, navigate post-treatment care, and optimize their health and well-being in the years following cancer treatment.

Late and Long-Term Effects of Treatment

Late and long-term effects of treatment for colon cancer may occur months or even years after completing treatment. These effects can vary depending on the type of treatment received, the individual's overall health, and other factors. Here are some common late and long-term effects of treatment for colon cancer:

Bowel Dysfunction: Surgery to remove part of the colon or rectum can result in changes in bowel function, such as diarrhea, constipation, urgency, or leakage (fecal incontinence). These symptoms may improve over time but can persist as long-term effects for some individuals.

Neuropathy: Chemotherapy drugs used to treat colon cancer, such as oxaliplatin, can cause nerve damage (peripheral neuropathy), resulting in symptoms such as numbness, tingling, pain, or weakness in the hands and feet. Neuropathy may improve after treatment but can sometimes become a chronic condition.

Fatigue: Fatigue is a common long-term effect of cancer treatment, including chemotherapy and radiation therapy. Some individuals may experience persistent fatigue even after completing treatment, which can impact daily functioning and quality of life.

Emotional and Psychological Effects: The emotional and psychological impact of colon cancer treatment can persist long after treatment ends. Survivors may experience anxiety, depression, fear of recurrence, post-traumatic stress symptoms, or changes in body image and self-esteem.

Cognitive Changes: Some individuals may experience cognitive changes or "chemo brain" following chemotherapy treatment, including difficulties with memory, concentration, attention, and multitasking. These cognitive changes can affect daily functioning and quality of life for some survivors.

Sexual Dysfunction: Treatment for colon cancer, including surgery, chemotherapy, and radiation therapy, can impact sexual function and intimacy. Survivors may experience changes in libido, erectile dysfunction (in men), vaginal dryness or discomfort (in women), and overall sexual satisfaction.

Infertility: Chemotherapy and radiation therapy can affect fertility in both men and women, potentially leading to temporary or permanent infertility. Individuals concerned about fertility preservation should discuss options with their healthcare provider before starting treatment.

Secondary Cancers: Some cancer treatments, such as radiation therapy and certain chemotherapy drugs, may increase the risk of developing secondary cancers later in life. Regular surveillance and follow-up care are important for monitoring for signs of secondary cancers.

Cardiovascular Effects: Certain chemotherapy drugs used to treat colon cancer, such as fluorouracil (5-FU) and capecitabine, may increase the risk of cardiovascular complications, including heart rhythm disturbances, cardiomyopathy, and ischemic heart disease.

Bone Health: Treatment for colon cancer, particularly hormone therapy or certain chemotherapy drugs, may impact bone health and increase the risk of osteoporosis or bone fractures. Adequate calcium and vitamin D intake, weight-bearing exercise, and bone density monitoring may be recommended to mitigate these risks.

It's important for cancer survivors to stay informed about potential late and long-term effects of treatment and to communicate openly with their healthcare providers about any symptoms or concerns that arise. Regular follow-up appointments and surveillance can help monitor for late effects, manage symptoms, and optimize overall health and well-being in the years following colon cancer treatment.

Recurrence: Signs, Symptoms, and Management

Recurrence of colon cancer refers to the return of cancer cells in the colon or rectum after a period of remission following initial treatment. Recognizing the signs and symptoms of recurrence and managing it promptly are essential for optimal outcomes. Here are some key points about recurrence, including signs, symptoms, and management:

Signs and Symptoms:

•Persistent or recurrent abdominal pain or discomfort

•Changes in bowel habits, such as new onset of constipation, diarrhea, or changes in stool consistency

•Blood in the stool or rectal bleeding

•Unexplained weight loss

•Fatigue or weakness

•Anemia (low red blood cell count)

•Obstruction of the colon or rectum, leading to symptoms such as cramping, bloating, or inability to pass stool or gas

•Jaundice (yellowing of the skin or eyes) if the cancer has spread to the liver

•New or worsening symptoms that persist despite conservative management

Diagnostic Tests:

•**Colonoscopy:** A colonoscopy may be performed to visualize the inside of the colon and rectum and to obtain biopsies of any suspicious lesions.

•**Imaging Studies:** Imaging tests such as CT scans, MRI scans, PET scans, or ultrasound may be used to detect the presence of cancer recurrence and assess its extent and location within the body.

•**Blood Tests:** Blood tests may be performed to measure tumor markers such as carcinoembryonic antigen (CEA), which may be elevated in individuals with recurrent colon cancer.

Management and Treatment:

•**Surgical Resection:** Depending on the location and extent of the recurrence, surgical resection may be considered to remove the recurrent tumor and any surrounding tissue. This may involve a partial colectomy or, in some cases, more extensive surgery.

•**Chemotherapy:** Chemotherapy may be recommended to treat recurrent colon cancer, either alone or in combination with surgery or radiation therapy. The specific chemotherapy regimen will depend on factors such as the individual's overall health, previous treatment history, and the characteristics of the recurrent cancer.

•**Radiation Therapy:** Radiation therapy may be used as part of the treatment plan for recurrent colon cancer, particularly if the cancer has spread to nearby structures or if surgery is not feasible.

•**Targeted Therapy:** Targeted therapy drugs, such as cetuximab or bevacizumab, may be used to treat recurrent colon cancer in individuals with specific genetic mutations or biomarker profiles.

•**Clinical Trials:** Participation in clinical trials may be an option for individuals with recurrent colon cancer, offering access to new and innovative treatment approaches that are not yet widely available.

Supportive Care: Supportive care measures may be implemented to help manage symptoms and improve quality of life for individuals with recurrent colon cancer. This may include palliative care, pain management, nutritional support, and psychosocial support services.

Regular Monitoring and Surveillance: After treatment for recurrent colon cancer, individuals will require regular monitoring and surveillance to monitor for any signs of further recurrence or progression of the disease. This may involve regular follow-up appointments, imaging studies, blood tests, and other tests as recommended by their healthcare provider.

Overall, early detection, prompt diagnosis, and appropriate management of recurrent colon cancer are crucial for optimizing outcomes and quality of life for affected individuals. It's important for individuals with a history of colon cancer to remain vigilant about monitoring for signs and symptoms of recurrence and to communicate openly with their healthcare providers about any concerns or changes in their health.

Advocacy and Resources for Patients and Survivors

Advocacy and resources for patients and survivors of colon cancer are essential for providing support, education, and empowerment throughout the cancer journey. Here are some key advocacy organizations and resources that individuals affected by colon cancer can turn to for support and assistance:

Colon Cancer Alliance (CCA): The Colon Cancer Alliance is a nonprofit organization dedicated to providing support, education, and advocacy for individuals affected by colon cancer. Their website offers a wealth of resources, including information about diagnosis, treatment, survivorship, and support services.

American Cancer Society (ACS): The American Cancer Society is a nationwide organization that provides support, resources, and advocacy for individuals affected by all types of cancer, including colon cancer. Their website offers information about colon cancer prevention, diagnosis, treatment, and support services, as well as opportunities for advocacy and volunteerism.

Fight Colorectal Cancer (Fight CRC): Fight Colorectal Cancer is a leading advocacy organization dedicated to raising awareness, funding research, and providing support for individuals affected by colorectal cancer. Their website offers resources, educational materials, and opportunities for advocacy and community engagement.

National Colorectal Cancer Roundtable (NCCRT): The National Colorectal Cancer Roundtable is a coalition of organizations committed to reducing the incidence and mortality of colorectal cancer through advocacy, education, and outreach. Their website offers resources for patients, survivors, healthcare providers, and advocates.

The Colon Club: The Colon Club is a nonprofit organization that provides support, advocacy, and education for young adults affected by colorectal cancer. Their website features personal stories, resources, and information about survivorship issues specific to young adults.

Online Support Communities: Online support communities and forums, such as CancerCare's online community or the Colorectal Cancer Support Group on Inspire, can provide a platform for individuals affected by colon cancer to connect with others, share experiences, and find support.

Local Support Groups: Many cancer centers, hospitals, and community organizations offer support groups for individuals affected by colon cancer. These support groups provide an opportunity to connect with others facing similar challenges, share information and resources, and receive emotional support.

Patient Advocacy Organizations: Patient advocacy organizations such as the Patient Advocate Foundation or Cancer Legal Resource Center can provide assistance with navigating insurance, financial issues, and legal matters related to cancer diagnosis and treatment.

Clinical Trial Matching Services: Clinical trial matching services, such as the American Cancer Society's Clinical Trials Matching Service or EmergingMed's TrialConnect, can help individuals find and access clinical trials for colon cancer treatment and research.

Educational Materials and Publications: Many advocacy organizations and healthcare providers offer educational materials, brochures, and publications about colon cancer prevention, diagnosis, treatment, and survivorship. These resources can help individuals and their families make informed decisions about their care.

By accessing these advocacy organizations and resources, individuals affected by colon cancer can find support, information, and assistance to navigate the challenges of diagnosis, treatment, survivorship, and beyond. Advocacy organizations play a crucial role in raising awareness, promoting early detection, advancing research, and improving outcomes for individuals affected by colon cancer.

Inspiring Stories of Survival

Stories of survival can provide hope, inspiration, and encouragement to individuals facing a diagnosis of colon cancer. Here are a few inspiring stories of survival from individuals who have overcome colon cancer:

Deborah Charles:

Deborah Charles was diagnosed with stage III colon cancer at the age of 38. Despite facing aggressive treatment, including surgery, chemotherapy, and radiation therapy, Deborah remained positive and determined throughout her journey. She used her experience to raise awareness about colon cancer and advocate for early detection and screening. Today, Deborah is a survivor and an advocate for others facing cancer.

Chris Draft:

Chris Draft, a former NFL player, lost his wife, Keasha, to colon cancer just one month after their wedding. Determined to honor her memory and raise awareness about the disease, Chris became a passionate advocate for colon cancer screening and prevention. He founded the Chris Draft Family Foundation to support cancer patients and promote healthy lifestyles. Despite the loss of his wife, Chris remains committed to making a difference in the fight against colon cancer.

Tom Marsilje:

Tom Marsilje, a cancer researcher and patient advocate, was diagnosed with stage IV colon cancer at the age of 45. Despite facing a grim prognosis, Tom became an outspoken advocate for cancer research and innovation. He used his scientific background to advocate for personalized treatment options and experimental therapies. Tom's resilience, positivity, and advocacy have inspired countless others in the cancer community.

Nalie Agustin:

Nalie Agustin was diagnosed with stage IV colon cancer at the age of 24. Determined to defy the odds and live life to the fullest, Nalie documented her cancer journey on social media, sharing her highs and lows with honesty and humor. She inspired thousands of followers with her resilience, positivity, and message of hope. Despite facing numerous setbacks, Nalie remains an advocate for cancer awareness and empowerment.

Colon Cancer Coalition Ambassadors:

The Colon Cancer Coalition features a diverse group of ambassadors who have survived colon cancer and are dedicated to raising awareness and supporting others facing the disease. These survivors share their stories, offer support and encouragement, and advocate for colon cancer screening and prevention in their communities.

These are just a few examples of the many inspiring stories of survival from individuals who have faced colon cancer with courage, determination, and resilience. Their stories remind us of the importance of early detection, screening, treatment, and support in the fight against colon cancer.

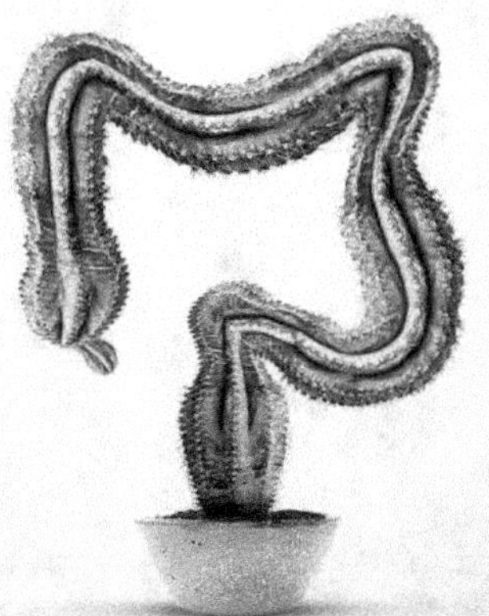

Colon cancer can run in families,
so if it's a concern, get screened early!
EARLY DETECTION IS KEY
In fighting this preventable disease.

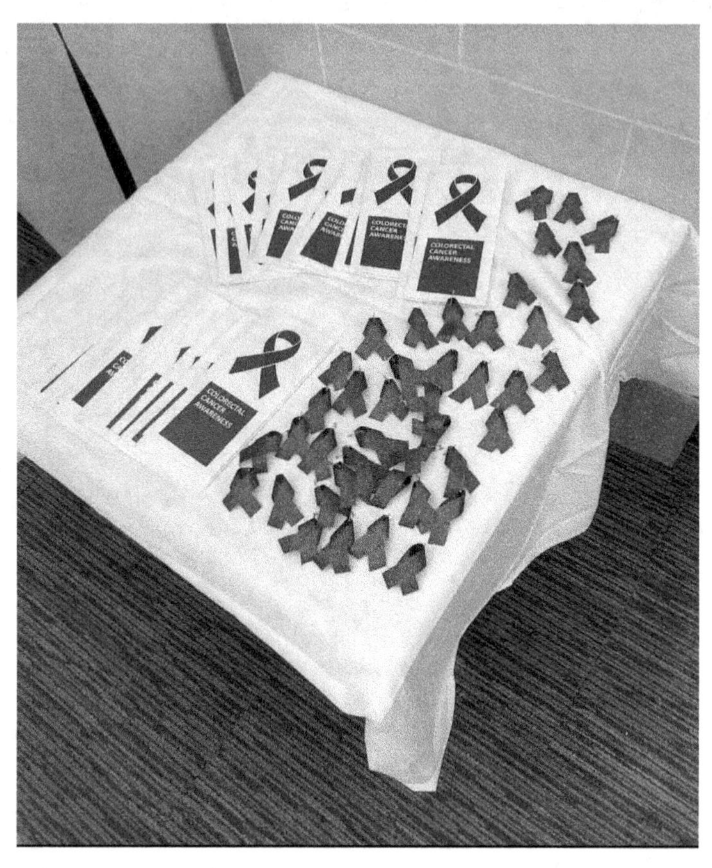

COLORECTAL CANCER AWARENESS

Conclusion

Hope and Future Directions in Colorectal Cancer Research

In conclusion, there is hope and optimism for the future of colorectal cancer research, diagnosis, treatment, and survivorship. Despite the challenges posed by this disease, significant progress has been made in recent years, leading to improved outcomes and quality of life for individuals affected by colorectal cancer. Here are some key points highlighting hope and future directions in colorectal cancer research:

Advances in Treatment: Advances in treatment modalities, including surgery, chemotherapy, radiation therapy, targeted therapy, and immunotherapy, have expanded treatment options and improved survival rates for individuals with colorectal cancer. Ongoing research continues to explore novel therapies and treatment strategies to further enhance outcomes and minimize side effects.

Precision Medicine: The emergence of precision medicine approaches, such as molecular profiling and genetic testing, has revolutionized the treatment of colorectal cancer by allowing for personalized, targeted therapies tailored to the individual's unique tumor characteristics and genetic makeup. Future research in this area holds promise for further advancements in precision oncology and individualized treatment approaches.

Immunotherapy: Immunotherapy, which harnesses the body's immune system to target and destroy cancer cells, has shown promising results in the treatment of colorectal cancer, particularly in individuals with microsatellite instability-high (MSI-H) tumors. Ongoing research aims to optimize immunotherapy strategies, identify biomarkers for patient selection, and overcome resistance mechanisms to enhance the efficacy of immunotherapy in colorectal cancer.

Early Detection and Screening: Early detection and screening remain critical in the fight against colorectal cancer, as early-stage disease is more treatable and associated with better outcomes. Research efforts are focused on developing non-invasive screening tests, improving existing screening modalities (such as colonoscopy and fecal occult blood testing), and increasing awareness and participation in screening programs to reduce the burden of colorectal cancer.

Biomarker Discovery: Research is underway to identify and validate novel biomarkers for colorectal cancer diagnosis, prognosis, and treatment response prediction. Biomarker discovery holds promise for improving early detection, guiding treatment decisions, and monitoring disease progression in individuals with colorectal cancer.

Prevention and Lifestyle Interventions: Research continues to explore the role of lifestyle factors, dietary habits, and environmental exposures in the development and prevention of colorectal cancer. Future studies will focus on identifying modifiable risk factors and developing targeted lifestyle interventions to reduce the incidence of colorectal cancer and improve overall population health.

Patient-Centered Care and Survivorship: There is increasing recognition of the importance of patient-centered care and survivorship support in colorectal cancer management. Future research will focus on addressing the psychosocial, emotional, and supportive care needs of individuals diagnosed with colorectal cancer, as well as improving access to survivorship care and resources to promote long-term health and well-being.

In summary, ongoing research efforts, technological advancements, and collaborative initiatives hold promise for further improving outcomes and quality of life for individuals affected by colorectal cancer. With continued dedication, innovation, and investment in research, there is optimism for a future where colorectal cancer is more effectively prevented, diagnosed, treated, and ultimately, overcome.

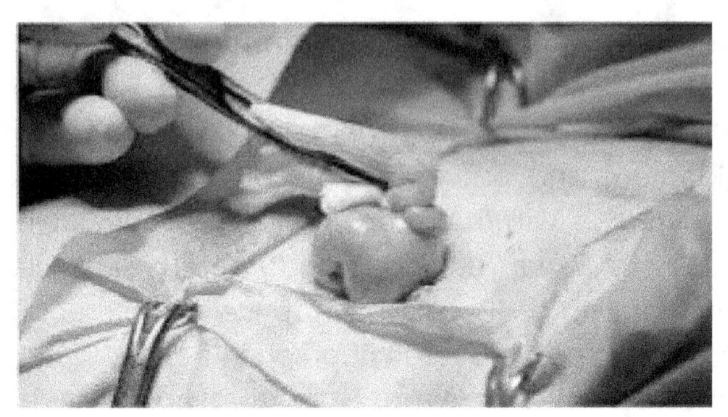

9 798320 072609